SUSAN DRURY

Tea Tree Oil

A Medicine Kit in a Bottle

SAFFRON WALDEN
THE C.W. DANIEL COMPANY LIMITED

First published in Australia
by Unity Press, Lindfield, NSW

This revised and up-dated edition
published in Great Britain in 1991
by the C.W. Daniel Company Limited
1 Church Path, Saffron Walden, Essex, CB10 1JP, England

ISBN 0 85207 238 4

Designed by Nevill Drury and Netan Pty Limited

Produced in association with
Book Production Consultants, Cambridge, England
Printed and bound by Clays Ltd., St. Ives plc

Foreword

THE BASIC MESSAGE about tea tree oil is that here we have one of the most marvellous healing resources that Nature has to offer. Here is an essential oil which has superb antiseptic qualities, which can treat burns, stings and skin irritations, which is invaluable for vaginal infections, tinea, arthritic pain, muscular aches and spasms, for infected gums and mouth ulcers — the list goes on and on . . .

Even more remarkable, perhaps, is the fact that tea tree oil is only now being rediscovered — for many years it has been neglected at the expense of the increasing scientific interest in synthetic medicines. Now we are beginning to realise that some of our most effective healing agents occur naturally and do not have to be concocted in a laboratory.

In 1925, the New South Wales government scientist Arthur Penfold announced an important discovery. He had just completed a three-year period of systematic testing and had found a species of tea tree — *Melaleuca alternifolia* — whose antiseptic properties were thirteen times stronger than carbolic acid, the main antibacterial weapon of the day. He also

noted that only the trees growing in the Bungawalbyn wetlands near Ballina in northern New South
Wales, had the appropriate medicinal concentration.

Penfold's findings stimulated further medical research and led to the establishment of around thirty
stills in and around the valley. The best tea tree oil
in the world still comes from this district — a relatively small area of 200 square kilometres.

The healing properties of tea tree oil were known
to the Bundjalung Aborigines and are far-ranging, as
indicated above. In addition to those applications,
tea tree oil can also be used for treating nasal congestion, boils, cold sores, sunburn, sore throats and a
number of fungal infections, including candidiasis.

The really amazing thing, it seems to me, is that
tea tree oil should have fallen into neglect for a
number of years. It was really because of the discovery of penicillin and the rise of antibiotics that tea
tree oil was forgotten. Since 1976, however, an Australian company call Thursday Plantation has been
busy replanting selected trees and redeveloping the
Bungawalbyn Creek region for the commercial dis-
tribution of tea tree oil. And in a move which must
have considerable impact on export potential, the
United States government has now approved the use
of tea tree oil in cosmetics. The oil can be used, for
example, not only in its pure state, but also as a con-
stituent in shampoos, soaps, antiseptic creams and
even in anti-itch treatments for pets! Even more recently, Thursday Plantation has secured approval to
sell its tea tree oil in Sweden, where strict government controls operate on therapeutics.

So tea tree oil is a very exciting substance indeed,
and one which — by all accounts — will soon find
a rapidly expanding world market.

This book presents, in a very readable and accessible way, not only the history and harvesting of tea tree oil but, even more importantly, an overview of its practical medical uses. It soon becomes obvious why we can label tea tree oil 'Nature's miracle healer'.

Nevill Drury
Editor, *Nature & Health*

Acknowledgments

Thanks are due to several individuals and organisations for information included in this book. These include Christopher Dean and Don Macdougall of Thursday Plantation; Christopher Beer, whose articles in *Nature & Health* were an especially valuable reference, and Dr Lyall Williams of the School of Chemistry, Macquarie University — who has also undertaken extensive research on the harvesting of tea tree oil.

Contents

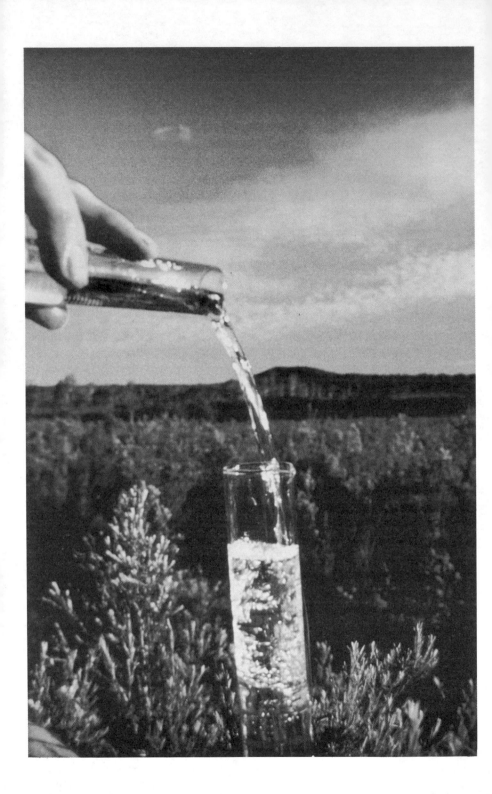

1

What is Tea Tree Oil?

TEA TREE OIL is the essence produced by distillation of the leaves of *Melaleuca alternifolia,* the medicinal tea tree. Its common name causes some confusion as the term 'tea tree' is widely used in Australia to describe a large group of shrubs and trees belonging to the two allied genera *Leptospermum* and *Melaleuca*, both of the family Myrtaceae. These plants are sometimes referred to as 'ti trees'. This spelling is incorrect. 'Ti' is the Maori name for a completely different tree, *Cordyline australis*, a palm-like plant from New Zealand commonly known as the cabbage tree.

The name 'tea tree' was first used by Captain Cook, whose sailors used the leaves of a species of Leptospermum as a substitute for tea. They found it 'spicy and refreshing'.

There are over three hundred varieties of tea tree widely spread throughout Australia and many of these produce essential oils with some healing properties. However, there is only one whose medicinal properties are outstanding. This is *Melaleuca alternifolia.*

This tree grows naturally on the north coast of New South Wales, particularly in the Richmond River basin near Lismore. It is quite difficult to distinguish from other species, particularly *Melaleuca linariifolia* which grows in an identical habitat. Some *Melaleuca alternifolia* trees can also be found near Newcastle and Sydney but, though they are botanically the same as the northern trees, their oils are very different. The trees from the north have a high terpinen-4-ol content and a low cineole content, while those from further south generally have a higher cineole content, so that the oil from trees in the Port Macquarie area resembles a cineole-rich eucalyptus oil. Cineole has useful medicinal qualities and is good for the relief of colds, but it is also a mucous membrane and skin irritant, so it is no good for healing wounds and inflammations.

In the early days of tea tree oil production it was very difficult to maintain quality control because some individual trees had much higher cineole content than others of the same species. This meant that oil from some trees, because of its high cineole content, could actually irritate the skin while the oil from other trees with a very low content of terpinen-4-ol had greatly reduced healing properties.

In 1948 three researchers, Penfold, Morrison and McKern, took a random sample of forty-nine trees from the north coast region of New South Wales and found that their cineole content varied between 6% and 16% of the total oil. The trees were botanically indistinguishable but their healing properties showed wide variations.

To establish some consistency in the quality of the oil it was decided that the trees should be classified according to their cineole content. Australian standard number AS 2782-1985 for Oil of Melaleuca now requires that the terpinen-4-ol content of the oil should be greater than 30% and the cineole content less than 15%. More recently the Australian Tea Tree Industry Association Inc. (ATTIA) has offered certification for oil which authentically meets the standard and comes only from *Melaleuca alternifolia*. It is important to buy only reputable brands to avoid unsatisfactory blends or even fraudulent concoctions which have been passed off as genuine tea tree oil.

Pure tea tree oil is colourless or sometimes pale yellow and has a pleasant characteristic smell. It is an extremely complex substance, containing at least 48 organic compounds. These consist mainly of terpinenes, cymones, pinenes, terpineols, cineol, sesquiterpenes and sesquiterpinene alcohols. Tea tree oil was the first natural substance found to contain the organic compound viridiflorene. A detailed analysis of the oil by Sword and Hunter (1978) revealed four constituents which have rarely been found anywhere else in Nature: viridiflorene (present at 1%), β terpineol (0.24%), L-terpineol (trace) and allyhexanoate (trace).

It is interesting to note that none of these substances is especially effective alone. It seems that all the compounds work together in synergy to produce the maximum healing power.

Recent studies undertaken by the Australian Tea Tree Industry Association (ATTIA) have determined the L.D. 50 or lethal dose in rats was 1.9–2.6 ml/kg. This oral toxicity parallels that found with other commonly used essential oils such as eucalyptus oil and suggests any internal use of the oil must be carefully supervised by a qualified practitioner. It is not advised that Tea Tree Oil be taken internally with the exception of occasional drops used for mouth ulcers, or gargled for sore throats.

Controlled studies have shown that Tea Tree Oil does not cause skin sensitisation problems and no obvious toxicity was observed even after prolonged skin contact trials.

Tea Tree Oil produced a negative result in the *in vitro* Ames screening test for carcinogenic potential indicating little or no carcinogenic hazard.

The potential for some skin irritation to occur in some people has been observed, and this seems to correlate with the concentration of oil used.

A correlation with better therapeutic qualities is found with the high terpinen-4-ol grades of Tea Tree Oil. This oil acts as a better bactericide and fungicide, while appearing to reduce the incidence of irritation. Oil with higher cineol and lower terpinen-4-ol is regarded as therapeutically inferior.

The trees which produce the finest quality of tea tree oil grow in the beautiful and remote swamp country around Bungawalbyn Creek near Ballina on the far north coast of New South Wales. This is where, in 1976, Thursday Plantation was established. Here the cultivation of only the finest trees ensures a regular supply of a consistently high quality oil. Independent laboratory tests of this oil have shown that it regularly displays a terpinen-4-ol concentration of more than 40% and a cineol content of less than 4%. The producers of this oil for the Ballinas company actually guarantee that their oil is above 36% terpinen-4-ol and below 7% cineol – the highest standard available. This means that oil from Thursday Plantation and the traditional tea tree forests around Bungawalbyn Creek is the best in the world.

While Australian Tea Tree Oil *(Melaleuca alternifolia)* has great applications in pure form, it is also available in a highly desirable miscible form containing 15% tea tree oil. This form has numerous benefits. It is milder to use, yet completely as effective as the concentrate. It is able to be readily mixed in water, so permitting a wide range of extra uses, and it is much more economical to use than the pure oil. In the directions for use of tea tree oil offered later in this book, the miscible form of the oil, at an active 15% level, is an ideal alternative to the pure concentrate in nearly all situations.

2

The History of Tea Tree Oil

FOR SOMETHING LIKE 40,000 years the Aboriginal people roamed peacefully over the Australian continent living in harmony with their natural environment. They killed animals and fish for food but did not engage in the sort of wholesale slaughter which threatened any species with extinction. They ate fruits and seeds from the trees and dug roots from the ground but managed to feed themselves without stripping the forests and laying waste to large areas of land. When they were sick or injured they generally managed to heal themselves without the help of modern drugs. They looked to the plants of the bush for their remedies and found a great number with strong medicinal properties.

Of course, the Aboriginal people did not classify their plants using the same categories and Latinised names as Linnaeus, nor did they record their remedies in old manuscripts. Much of the medicinal knowledge possessed by many Aboriginal tribes has died with the destruction of the rest of their culture, but fortunately some of the early settlers were sufficiently observant to notice the remedies used by the

Aboriginal people living in their area. The more open-minded even tried them out themselves, often with surprisingly effective results.

The Bundjalung Aborigines who lived in north-eastern New South Wales around Bungawalbyn Creek were well aware of the amazing healing qualities of the tea trees which abounded in the swampy areas. They treated their cuts and wounds and any kind of skin infection by crushing the leaves of the tea tree, sprinkling them liberally over the injury and then covering it with a warm mud pack.

Later the white men came in search of 'red gold', the highly prized tall cedar of the rainforest. They were too far away from their own doctors to rely on any European medicines so they used what was available locally and were surprised how well it worked. As new settlers came to the area they battled to clear the land of its native vegetation to open it up for the newly developing dairy industry. While they cursed the tea tree plants for their tenacious grip on the land and sweated over the exhausting process of grubbing out the roots of the plant by hand, they were still happy to use its healing leaves for any injuries or infection.

For many years tea tree oil was a popular, well recognised natural antiseptic. It was not until the development of synthetically manufactured commercial drugs that the natural oil began to be regarded as something of an old wives' remedy and people preferred to put their faith in pills obtained with a doctor's prescription.

Today the situation is reversed. Many people have become disillusioned with modern synthetic drugs and worried about their potentially harmful side-effects. There is a worldwide trend back to 'natural' remedies and tea tree oil is enjoying a great resurgence in popularity. It is available in health food shops and from chemists all over the country, and is also recognised in other parts of the world.

The scientific community has also shown considerable interest in the oil of *Melaleuca alternifolia*. Sir Joseph Banks collected samples of tea tree leaves when he travelled to Australia with Captain Cook in 1770 but he seems to have been unaware of the potential healing properties of his specimens and for a long time tea tree oil remained a bush remedy known only to the Aborigines and to a handful of white settlers living in the north-eastern corner of New South Wales.

Then, in the early 1920s, Arthur Penfold, *FCS*, an astute government chemist who worked as the curator and economic chemist at the Museum of Technology and Applied Sciences in Sydney, began to undertake some very interesting work. He had noticed the very high antiseptic power of tea tree oil and in 1922 began a series of laboratory experiments. In 1925 he announced his results. Tea tree oil had been shown to have antiseptic qualities thirteen times stronger than carbolic acid, the accepted standard of the time. It had the added advantage of being non-toxic and non-irritating. This astounding discovery lead to much enthusiastic research.

By 1930 the *Medical Journal of Australia* featured an article headed 'A New Australian Germicide'. It reported the pleasing results gained in general practice by applying tea tree oil to septic wounds, carbuncles and pus-filled infections and stated: 'The results obtained in a variety of conditions when it was first tried were most encouraging, a striking feature being that it dissolved pus and left the surfaces of infected wounds clean, so that its germicidal action became more effective without any apparent damage to the tissues. This was something new, as most efficient germicides destroy tissue as well as bacteria.'

The article particularly recommended tea tree oil for 'dirty wounds such as are frequently seen as the result of street accidents' and noted that the pus solvent properties of tea tree oil made it an excellent lotion for 'perionchia' (paronychia) which, if untreated, frequently results in the loss or deformity of the nails. Infections like this, which had resisted treatment for months, had been cleaned up in less than a week after regular application of tea tree oil.

Mr E Morris Humphery, the author of the article, also noted that two drops of tea tree oil in a tumbler of warm water made an excellent gargle to clear up sore throats in the early stages, and suggested that tea tree oil would probably be good for other infections of the naso-pharynx. He found the pleasant smelling oil was an excellent deodorant and immediately cleared away any foul smell from a wound or abscess. If added to ordinary hand soap its action on typhoid bacilli was found to be more than sixty times as rapid as other so-called disinfectant soaps. Humphery felt, too, that an ointment made from tea tree oil would be an excellent treatment for several parasitic skin diseases.

The medical world was very impressed by the claims made for the humble Australian tree. More research was done and articles appeared in journals such as *The Medical Journal of Australia*, *The Australian Journal of Pharmacy* and *The Australian Journal of Dentistry*. In 1930 an Australian dentist wrote an article for the August issue of his professional journal. He stated:

> 'Our choice of antiseptics in work about the mouth
> is all-important, and much of the success of treat-
> ment will depend upon correct choice and correct
> use of them.
>
> When I see men advocating the use of drugs in
> pus-forming conditions in the oral cavity without
> any thought for their destructive action upon the
> tissues involved, I wish they would realise that they
> are simply lowering the natural defence and creat-
> ing an excellent pabulum for the development of
> the next crop of bacteria.
>
> We have many excellent antiseptics at hand
> which will play their part and help Nature to take
> the active role in repair work that she is ever ready
> to take, do we but give her the opportunity. Let me
> remind you that the ideal to be sought in an anti-
> septic is that it is:-
>
> **1** Of high antiseptic power
>
> **2** Non-irritating to tissue cells
>
> **3** Non-toxic
>
> Many drugs of value to us in our work do not
> possess these combined uses and they must there-
> fore be used in free dilution and sparingly . . .
>
> During the last three months I have been trying
> out a product of our own Australian trees, a new
> essential oil discovered by Mr W. R. Penfold, at the
> Technological Museum, Sydney, and tested and re-
> ported upon by Dr E. Morris Humphery, of Sydney
> (*A.M.J.* March 29, 1930). Mr Penfold's analysis
> showed it to be non-toxic, non-irritating, and 11 to
> 13 times stronger than carbolic as a germicide
> (Rideal-Walker coefficient).

This and Dr Humphery's report of cases appealed so strongly to me that I made a special request for some of the oil to try out for mouth work. As the raw product it has been called Ti-trol, and in soluble form, Melasol. It is obtained in Northern districts of New South Wales and Queensland from a species of Tea-tree, the *Melaleuca alternifolia*, and prepared by the Australian Essential Oil Co., Sydney.

After trying out in several tests, I feel confident that in Ti-trol and Melasol we have an antiseptic which more nearly answers the ideal than any I have previously tested for our special work and in general surgery it should be of even greater value.'

The interest was not confined to Australia. News of this exciting healing oil spread to other countries of the world and was presented in articles in the *Journal of the National Medical Association* (USA) and the *British Medical Journal*, which stated in 1933 that 'the oil is a powerful disinfectant but is non-poisonous and non-irritant, and has been used successfully in a very wide range of septic conditions.'

As its reputation spread, many people were tempted to try tea tree oil as a last resort, after other treatments had failed. There is a great deal of anecdotal evidence about its effectiveness. In 1936 an aqueous suspension of the oil was successfully used to clear up a very severe case of diabetic gangrene. The sailors aboard *HMS Sussex* were saved considerable discomfort when their surgeon-lieutenant applied tea tree oil to the feet of the dozens of crew members who had developed tinea while their ship was stationed at the port of Alexandria in Egypt.

Tea tree oil was even used on animals. The November issue of *Poultry* in 1936 recommended the use of Ti-trol to prevent cannibalism in poultry. It stated that injuries treated with Ti-trol healed much more quickly and that the smell seemed to ward off attacks by other chooks in the cage.

During the 1930s the oil of *Melaleuca alternifolia*, then known as Ti-trol or, in aqueous solution as Melasol, became a scientifically recognised treatment used successfully around the world by dentists for pyorrhoea, gingivitis, nerve-capping and haemorrhages. It was used by doctors for throat infections, gynaecological conditions and all sorts of dirty or pus-filled infections and had also been shown to have a remarkable effect on a wide range of skin fungi, including tinea, candida and parionychia.

Demand for this excellent oil was far greater than supply. Commercial production was really only at the small cottage industry level. All harvesting was done by hand by expert cutters who stripped the trees of their leaves using lightweight razor sharp machetes. They worked only on trees growing in their natural habitat — often deep in fairly inaccessible swampy bushland. When the cutters returned with their hessian bags full of leaves the latter were tipped into pots of water and boiled over slow-burning log fires.

Although there were at one time up to thirty stills in the Bungawalbyn area, none produced oil on a very large scale, the quality was not always consistent and, if floods or other difficulties prevented the cutters from harvesting a sufficient number of leaves, then their production levels could not be met.

One of the earliest pioneers of the new commercial tea tree oil industry was Mr H. James, managing director of Australian Essential Oils Ltd. By 1929 this company had established an early lead in the industry by securing access to extensive areas of natural stands along Bungawalbyn Creek, a tributary of the Richmond River near Coraki. Once he was confident he could obtain sufficient supplies from the wild *Melaleuca alternifolia* he formulated a water miscible product which he called 'Melasol' and then arranged for leading medical and dental practitioners to conduct valuable fundamental research into the properties and medical applications of the oil, which he called Ti-trol, and also of the aqueous solution.

In 1936 Australian Essential Oils published a report summarising the reactions of the various medical practitioners who had used oil of Melaleuca in the early 1930s. Many of them tried this natural product only after more orthodox remedies had proved unsuccessful, so this made their results even more remarkable. The doctors and dentists were impressed by both products but noticed some differences in their action. They observed that the pure oil (Ti-trol) had greater penetration where there was no free moisture and so penetrated unbroken skin more effectively than the water miscible form. On the other hand, Melasol mixed better with tissue, pus and membrane where they were exposed by broken skin, inflammation or internal cavities.

It is very interesting to note that the authors of the report state: 'There has been no large organisation working to build up a presentable superstructure of tests to create a new market, but the results are due to the co-operation of a large number of practitioners who have no commercial interest in the company.' Apparently tea tree oil needed no promoting. The quality of the results spoke for itself.

By the time the Second World War broke out, tea tree oil was considered such an essential commodity that cutters and producers were exempted from war service. All stocks of tea tree oil were taken over for the war effort and tea tree oil was taken off its developing market place for several years in a row. The government hoped to accumulate sufficient supplies of this precious essence so that it could be supplied as standard issue in all army and navy first-aid kits in tropical regions. Large quantities of the oil of *Melaleuca alternifolia* were incorporated in machine-cutting oils to reduce infections from skin injuries, especially abrasions to the hands by metal filings and turnings.

However, the producers found it impossible to keep up sufficient supplies of tea tree oil. Scientific researchers had developed some synthetically made alternative germicides and, though these were not as effective as the natural oil, they were available in much larger quantities so they soon replaced the natural product. After the war ended the pure oil of *Melaleuca alternifolia* was almost impossible to buy. The market was flooded with an increasing number of synthetically produced 'miracle drugs', such as penicillin, and most people were quite confident that man could improve upon Nature. Old remedies were cast aside in favour of 'modern' and 'scientifically developed' chemicals.

By the early 1950s there were only three stills operating near the Bungawalbyn Valley. However, two decades later the situation began to look quite different. As a flow on from the 'hippie' revolution of the 1960s many people began to be disillusioned with some aspects of modern society and began to be concerned about the possible side-effects of the powerful drugs prescribed by so many doctors. They became aware, too, of the pollution of the environ-

ment caused by such widespread use of manufactured chemicals. Scientists began to observe that
man-made antibiotics were no longer as effective in
treating disease and that some organisms were developing a resistance to their effects. People were increasingly disillusioned with modern science.
'Natural' products came back into vogue and the
time was right for the rediscovery of natural tea tree
oil.

One of the reasons tea tree oil has never been
available in very large quantities is that the oil has all
come from trees growing wild in the bush. These
trees grow naturally in only one part of the world,
scattered in remote parts of a small area of about
200 square kilometres in the north-eastern corner of
New South Wales. Their swampy habitat is prone to
floods and harvesting is often difficult.

In 1976 a new development occurred in the tea
tree industry which was to change its character completely. Christopher Dean, an honours graduate in
Social Anthropology and a former social worker
from Sydney, decided to give up his city life and
settle on the north coast. It was a very well considered move. He and his father spent six years getting
to know the land around Bungawalbyn Creek and
learning the secrets of growing tea trees. For five
years Christopher and his wife Lynda lived with
their three young children in a small tractor shed
without power, telephone or neighbours. Two of
their children were born at home, in this tiny
wooden cabin.

The Deans were attempting something that had
never been tried before. They were deliberately set-
ting up a tea tree farm from which oil could be produced on a commercial scale. This meant they

planted only specially selected trees — ones whose oil had been proven to be of the highest quality. It meant, too, that they could plant trees in positions where they could be more easily harvested. For the first time it appeared possible that Australia might be able to realise the commercial possibilities of tea tree oil.

In the early days of his work on the tea tree plantation Christopher Dean might well have been tempted to abandon the whole project. Like all pioneers he suffered from a number of setbacks and the process of learning by trial and error was often a discouraging one. However, he did have a personal belief in the healing qualities of the oil he was cultivating and was determined to make this miracle oil available to others.

Christopher had spent some months in Africa in the early 1970s and had developed an infectious fungus under his toenails. He had tried all the usual and many unusual remedies without success and the fungus continued to spread. When he finally reached London he sought the attention of a medical specialist who could see no other solution except having the toenail removed and the offending skin cut off with the risk of permanent damage to the foot. Fortunately Christopher's brother arrived in London the next day and had with him the bottle of tea tree oil he always carried when travelling. They decided this simple natural remedy was well worth a try, so they applied it to Christopher's foot. Within four days the infection had cleared completely!

Here was yet another successful story to encourage the Dean family in their interest in the oil of *Melaleuca alternifolia*. Christopher Dean's stepfather, Mr Eric White, had been engaged in research on the tea tree oil industry for many years. He worked closely with Brian Small of the New South Wales Department of Agriculture, who directly supported and encouraged him. Eventually, one auspicious Thursday, the Deans were granted a lease of Crown land to establish a commerical tea tree plantation. Its name, of course, was to be Thursday Plantation.

At first Christopher and his wife distilled only very small quantities of oil and freely distributed it to friends. They were so impressed that the Deans decided to set up a stall at the Sunday markets. These markets are a very important institution among the 'alternative' people on the north coast of New South Wales. Each Sunday thousands of people — both locals and tourists — wander in to enjoy a pleasant social occasion. There is home-made food, entertainment for the children, and music from anyone who feels in the mood for performing. Stall holders sell almost anything — organically grown fruit and vegetables, locally made handicrafts, imported 'ethnic' jewellery, second hand clothes and herbal remedies. The tea tree oil from the Dean's farm was an enormous success and health food shops in the area began stocking the oil for those who did not manage to get to the markets. The Deans were unable to keep up the supply. Soon a local man called 'Snow', who had worked as a tea tree cutter for fifteen years, began to supply leaf on a contract basis to Thursday Plantation. Others in the area followed his example — some working full-time and others using it as a weekend job to earn a bit more money. Some leaves are of higher quality than others so the cutters were paid for the oil distilled from their leaves — at the then rate of about $16 per litre.

Within a few years, health stores and pharmacies all over Australia were selling the Dean's oil, which they successfully marketed as 'a medicine kit in a bottle'. At the present time demand for the oil is still greater than the amount which can be supplied. A new plantation is being planted in the Ballina district with all the knowledge gained from past experience and using upgraded plant varieties which have been designed to meet specific market needs.

As well as pure tea tree oil, it is now possible to buy tea tree antiseptic cream. This is a water-based emolient cream with 5% oil. It is used for a variety of skin irritations and has the advantage of being easier to apply. Tea tree oil is also available as a high quality skin-care soap. The oil has a high boiling point and retains its stability when blended with soap. Because it is so gentle in its action on the skin, relatively high proportions can be added without causing skin irritation. Soap containing 4% tea tree oil has a germicidal value sixteen times greater than the carbolic soap so widely used in the 1930s. The soap produced by Thursday Plantation contains 2% tea tree oil, which makes it a very effective agent for treating acne and other skin infections. Thursday Plantation has also incorporated tea tree oil into a range of shampoos and conditioners which have been well received by the public.

As its popularity increases, market analysts have estimated that world demand for tea tree oil could reach 700 tonnes per annum by 1998. In 1985 only 10 tonnes were produced, so obviously there is much room for expansion. Production in 1990 exceeded 60 tonnes.

The success of Thursday Plantation has encouraged new people to join the industry. With varying degrees of success, plantations have been set up in a number of different areas such as Nambucca, Taree, and even as far south as Hornsby, a Sydney suburb which has a climate quite different from the trees' original habitat.

Many millions of dollars have been invested in tea tree growing to bring this 'Aussie Gold' onto the world market. The United States government has now approved oil of *Melaleuca alternifolia* for use in cosmetics and the way is open for this humble tree to become a giant export earner for Australia.

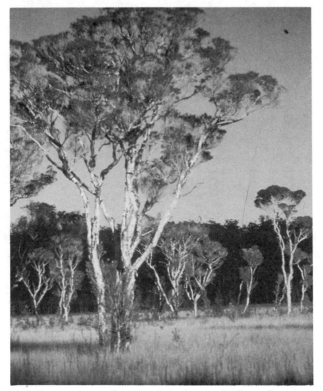

A fully grown tea tree stands in front of a large forest. Trees are invigorated by the harvesting.

3
Harvesting The Oil

MELALEUCA ALTERNIFOLIA, from which this amazing oil is obtained, is a paper-bark tree with narrow feathery leaves of a bright fresh green colour. It does not usually grow above about six metres tall. White settlers on the north coast of New South Wales have long regarded it as a pest and have laboured to clear it out and to drain the swamps in which it grows so that the land can be used for cattle, sugar cane or other crops. At a time when Australia's sugar and dairy industries are becoming increasingly less profitable, it is ironical to look at the money which could have been made by selling tea tree oil if the land had been left in its natural state. Dairy farmers have always regarded the tea tree as a particular nuisance because it is almost impossible to kill except by digging out all the roots. Even if all the branches are cut off and the tree reduced to a stump, new shoots will appear with surprising rapidity and the tree soon resumes its normal size.

For the producers of tea tree oil this quality has been the tree's greatest asset. Until very recently there has been no need to go to the trouble and expense of actually planting trees. The cutters needed only to follow their customary tracks through the bush, strip all trees of their branches, and return with their rich harvest. Because the work was hard and the trees fairly difficult to get to, by the time a cutter had worked his way through all the trees in his area, the original ones would be covered in luxuriant new growth and the whole process could start again.

This was an excellent method of harvesting. No damage occurred to the trees or to the natural ecosystem and the regular pruning actually stimulated the new growth. The trees along the Bungawalbyn Creek which have been harvested regularly for over sixty years are recognised to be the healthiest and most vigorous found anywhere. This is in marked contrast to man's usual agricultural activities which often involve draining the soil of its nutrients so they have to be replaced by chemical fertilisers, or clearing large areas of country of their natural vegetation and so leaving the land vulnerable to the effects of soil erosion.

Most of the older tree cutters have a special rapport with the land. They feel a deep love of the bush and, though their work is arduous and requires great physical stamina and skill, they enjoy the solitary life and the feeling of being perfectly attuned to the environment. While other workers must put up with the noise of machinery, the din of traffic and the constant pressure of people all around, the old tea tree cutters spend their days deep in the stillness of the forest where the quiet is broken only by the calls of the native birds or the rustle of falling leaves in the thick vegetation.

The working day starts very early for these old-timers, as it does for most country people. At first glimmer of dawn the cutters set out, carrying only a supply of large hessian bags and a light weight, razor-sharp machete which is a modified martindale cane knife. Many of the trees are accessible only on foot. There are some specially adapted 4-wheel drive vehicles used to reach the natural stands of leaf but they often get bogged in the mud. This is an area of high rainfall and, as anyone who has visited the north coast will know, the rain here is quite different from the gentle drizzle of the south. The skies literally seem to fall open and the rain buckets down, drenching the land and the people below. Often the soil is already saturated so there is nowhere for the water to run. It therefore lies around in large pools till it is eventually dried up by the scorching sun. The people who live on the north coast are used to sudden flash floods and have managed to adapt to them — so too must the tea tree harvesters. They must do without the mechanical aids which have taken the drudgery out of much modern agriculture.

Harvesting tea tree is not an easy job. The suckers are cut off the stumps and each branch is stripped individually with the cane knife. The best cutters will strip nearly one tonne of leaves in a day by grasping the branches in one hand, holding them upside down, and then slashing with the knife. Good cutters work with unbelievable speed. Needless to say, they cannot afford even the tiniest slip in concentration.

The leaves are then loaded into hessian bags and taken back to the still. Each leaf has a number of tiny sacs which contain the precious essential oil. If the leaf is crushed these glands break open and release the strongly smelling vapour. It is interesting to note that modern producers still use the traditional method of distilling this oil in an old-fashioned, wood-fired, steam distillation unit. The leaves and terminal branches of the tree are emptied into large vats, called pots. Water is boiled with slow-burning log fires and the steam passes up through the leaves, bursting the capillaries on each leaf and releasing the oil vapour from the hundreds of minute glands on each leaf. The steam and oil vapour are then channelled through a long metal coil immersed in cold water — the condenser. The now liquid oil passes through a collection tank where the oil floats to the surface and is siphoned off and filtered. Each still holds approximately one tonne of leaf material and will usually yield around 1 per cent, or 10 litres of clear to pale yellow oil with a distinctive spicy aroma.

After filtering, each batch of tea tree oil is carefully analysed to check that the chemical composition satisfies the Australian standard requirements and to meet rigid quality control specifications. It must have a terpinen-4-ol content of at least 30 per cent and a cineole content of less than 15 per cent. Many of the better quality oils reach even higher standards than these but not all oil from the bush trees is of consistently high quality.

Modern Plantations

In 1988 the majority of Australian tea tree oil still came from individual bush cutters who collected the leaves from the prolific natural stands of *Melaleuca alternifolia* along the swamps and water courses of northern New South Wales. The trees grow very well here and it has often been assumed that this is their natural habitat and they would not thrive anywhere else. However, there is also the possibility that they grow in swampy, inaccessible areas mainly because these areas are not suitable for anything else. The better quality land has already been cleared and used for dairy cattle or, more recently, for more exotic crops like avocados or macadamia nuts — or even for new housing estates. Several trial plots have shown that, with appropriate cultivation, weed control and adequate water supply, *Melaleuca alternifolia* will grow better than it does in poor swampy soil.

The same sort of discovery was made about Jojoba. The natural habitat of this plant is in the Sonora Desert in the United States of America. When its healing properties became well known, several entrepreneurs tried to harvest it and hoped for substantial profits but they found it was not a commercial success. However, it was soon discovered that jojoba would grow much better on good quality soil with more regular water. A plantation near Rockhampton in Queensland produced a small crop after only its second year of cultivation, something which is unheard of in the plant's arid native habitat.

Similarly, Christopher Dean at Thursday Plantation and several other Australian companies are experimenting with the idea of growing *Melaleuca alternifolia* on better quality soil to see if this will improve the yield of oil. There seem to be several advantages in establishing plantations of specially selected trees. In the 1930s and 1940s it looked as though production of tea tree oil would become a flourishing Australian industry. People all over the world were very impressed with the healing qualities of the oil, yet the producers of tea tree oil found it very difficult to make a steady profit.

Mrs Tod Berry who, with her husband, took over the most successful of the companies, Australian Essential Oils (later known as Pacific Manufacturing), explained that 'the eventual decline of tea tree oil was due to several factors such as unreliable supply, inconsistent quality and most importantly, lack of promotion.' When she retired in 1975 her company was sold and all records dealing with tea tree oil, its history and medical applications, were apparently destroyed.

It is a truism that young entrepreneurs are always confident of success where others have failed. While Christopher Dean and other producers continued to rely on oil from native bush stands they would be handicapped by the sorts of problems which faced earlier producers. However, once they had the idea of establishing new plantations the situation began to look entirely different.

For anyone considering the establishment of a new plantation the first problem is that of obtaining young plants of good quality stock. Different companies have gone about this in different ways. Some have chosen to plant seeds collected from trees in stands which have been shown to produce high quality oil. This is not necessarily a reliable method because in the plantation the oil yield, per hectare, per annum, will be determined by the amount of oil in the leaves and also by the rate of biomass production. Trees in their natural state will not necessarily grow in the same way as those under plantation conditions.

A recent study at Macquarie University, Sydney, revealed large differences in the size of trees produced from seed. Some trees were tall and had a single trunk, others were short and bushy and had a much greater biomass. When seedlings which had been planted in October 1985 were harvested twelve months later (in October 1986) they had an average biomass of 0.65 kg per tree. Those seedlings which were allowed to grow for fifteen months (till January 1987) before harvesting had an average biomass of 1.6 kg. However, some individual trees had already developed a biomass of 2.5 times this weight (4 kg).

It is obvious that the industry will be much more profitable if seedlings are well chosen so that they all develop into trees with a larger than average biomass. Much further research is needed in this area.

Another difficulty is the minute size of the seeds. Seeds of *Melaleuca alternifolia* are so tiny they look like very finely ground pepper and it takes about 40,000 of them to make up 1 gram. Some companies such as Condux Industries grow the seeds in separate containers and then eventually plant them out in the field. This method is expensive and labour-intensive but has a high rate of success.

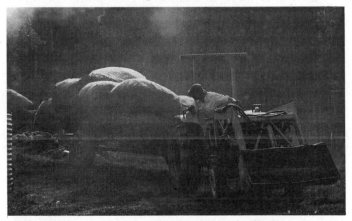

The cutters unload the bagged leaf into the still. The traditional distillation technology is simple and safe.

Another company, Australian Tea Tree Estates, distributes the seeds over the soil in grow-tunnels which are covered with clear plastic film and fitted with misting sprays to maintain hot and humid conditions to help the seeds to grow. Once the seedlings are about 30 cm tall they are planted out by mechanical harvesting equipment. The plants are gently washed to remove the propagating medium and disentangle the roots, and are then placed in containers partly filled with water and transferred to the planting machine. This is a rotating wheel with a number of carrier arms which places each seedling into a furrow, presses it down, and then releases it. This is certainly the cheapest method of planting but unless planting conditions are perfect many seedlings suffer from plant shock and die.

Some of the finer roots that absorb water and nutrient are lost when using this method — commonly known as the bare root method — so it is essential to keep the plant and surrounding soil moist for at least the first week to minimise transplant shock. A well established tea tree may be hard to eradicate but in the early stages it is very vulnerable.

It has been suggested that selected trees should be propagated by cuttings instead of by seed selection. This would be a more reliable method of ensuring the young trees had the same characteristics and would ensure a population of superior trees.

Spacing of Trees

Tea tree planting is a new kind of agriculture and a great deal of research and experimentation must be undertaken before growers can determine even such basic matters as how far apart the trees should be planted and what is the best space to leave between rows. In its natural habitat *Melaleuca alternifolia* grows in very dense bush. This makes harvesting extremely difficult as the work has to be done by hand. No machinery can operate in such a restricted space and the land is so swampy that all vehicles get bogged.

At first, producers thought that the planting of trees in well spaced rows would make harvesting much easier and of course it does. However, research such as that by Small (1981) has shown that plants may produce more leaf per hectare when they are very close together. Several new commercial plantations have chosen densities of 20–25,000 plants per hectare. This seems at the present time to be the optimum concentration. Only time and further experimentation will tell whether this is the case.

Harvesting

Melaleuca alternifolia is quite a fast-growing tree. In the first year it produces one or two trunks which, depending on soil and climatic conditions, may attain heights of up to two metres. Some trees are ready for their first harvesting only twelve to fifteen months after they have been planted. When the trunks are cut, the regrowth consists of multiple shoots sprouting from the side of the base so that the plant looks more like a bush than a tree.

Special harvesters are now being used to cut the trees above the ground and then transfer the leaves and branches to the still where they will be processed by the traditional method of steam distillation.

Most farmers are in little doubt about the correct

time to harvest their crops. Years of experience have taught them that pawpaws picked while they are still too green will never attain the same full flavour as those which have been allowed to ripen on the tree. On the other hand, peaches or plums left on the tree till they are ready to be eaten will arrive in the city bruised and rotting. Most tea tree growers do not yet have this experience, and research is still being undertaken to determine the optimum time for harvesting.

Seasoned bush cutters have always noticed that both the quality and the quantity of oil fluctuates according to the season in which the leaves are cut. Penfold and his co-workers reported 'the oil yield is lower in winter months than in summer, a sudden increase appearing in November, the first month of summer, the yield falling off again about June, the first winter month in northern New South Wales.' (Penfold, Morrison and McKern, 1948)

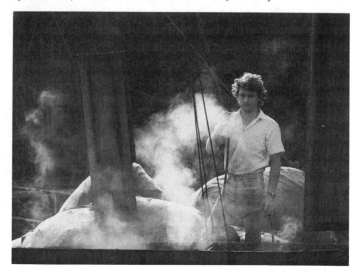

They fill the still to the top. A good cutter will bring a ton of leaf from the bush each day.

For commerical growers the situation is a little more complicated. When deciding the optimum time for harvesting they must consider not only the total biomass and amount of oil present in the leaf at the time but also the speed with which the tree will regrow. Research is being undertaken at Macquarie University (Williams and Home, 1987) to try to give growers more information in these areas but it is not yet conclusive. It seems that not all trees reach their maximum oil content at the same time and variations in rainfall cause further fluctuations in oil yield. It has been tentatively suggested that harvesting could commence in December and continue till June, and that trees cut earlier in the summer will have a higher rate of regrowth and so increase the harvest for the following year. No doubt it will take several more years of trial and error before tea tree growers can feel confident that their farming practices are ensuring the maximum yield of oil is obtained from their trees.

4

Health Uses

Acne and Pimples

ACNE IS AN extremely common skin condition, generally caused by hormonal changes which lead to an increase in the activity of the sebaceous glands of the face, chest and back. The sebum produced becomes trapped beneath the skin, forming a plug often called a blackhead. When this becomes infected it forms a pimple.

Doctors generally agree there is no miracle cure for acne and that in most cases it will eventually disappear. This is no consolation for the thousands of teenagers who feel their social life is being ruined by unsightly pimples and who spend a great deal of money trying the latest well-advertised acne lotion. Most skin specialists agree that acne sufferers should avoid rich fatty foods and eat plenty of fresh fruit and vegetables, and they stress the importance of washing with a good antiseptic soap and exposing the face to sunlight (for a short time). Handling the face or squeezing pimples will often cause them to spread, so this should be avoided.

There are a large number of proprietory lotions and creams for acne. Many of these do do some good as they all have antiseptic qualities which help to stop the spread of infection. However, some of them are very harsh, often peroxide-type bleaches and, if applied freely, can irritate the healthy skin, especially in the sensitive parts of the face. This is the great advantage of tea tree oil. It is a very strong antiseptic but because its cineol content is so low, it is quite soothing and does not harm the delicate skin of the face[1].

Because it has the unusual ability to penetrate beneath the surface of the skin it can help to clear up 'blind' pimples which often take so long to heal.

There is, as yet, no clinical evidence to support the use of tea tree oil for acne but there are a great many individuals who have tried dabbing the oil onto their pimples and have found the results almost miraculous. The usual method is to wash the face well and then apply tea tree oil with the finger or a cotton bud directly from the bottle three or four times the first day, then two or three times a day for the next three days. An alternative is to add three to six drops of the pure oil to warm water and rinse the face thoroughly.

Tea tree oil is also available in an attractively packaged fresh yellow soap with a pleasant, tangy smell. This soap contains 2 per cent of oil of *Melaleuca alternifolia* and is a useful aid in the treatment of acne, even for the most sensitive skins. Thursday Plantation also produces a non-greasy Antiseptic Cream which can be applied to the face to treat acne.

[1] See also page 83, *New Findings on Acne*

Arthritis

THIS IS AN inflammation of the tissues of one or more joints, which usually causes pain and swelling. It has a number of different causes and may be either acute (often following an injury or infection) or chronic. The two most common forms of chronic arthritis are rheumatoid arthritis, which may occur in young people and osteoarthritis, which usually occurs in the elderly. Both forms are usually treated by analgesics and anti-inflammatory drugs.

Some people find relief from arthritic pains by mixing three to five drops of tea tree oil into a small amount of baby oil and massaging it deeply into the joints. Tea tree oil has the special property of being able to penetrate through the skin to work on the tissue beneath, and its mildly anaesthetic qualities give relief from the pain.

Boils and Abscesses

AN ABSCESS IS a local pocket of infection. In the skin, where it often starts around a hair follicle, it is known as a boil. Usually a boil begins as a small, painful swelling; the follicle and surrounding cells are killed by bacteria and after two or three days form a core of pus under the skin. Eventually the boil comes to a head and the pus bursts through the skin and escapes. Some particularly unfortunate people develop carbuncles, which are actually collections of boils. They form when more than one hair follicle becomes infected. Channels of pus may be extensive and spread below the skin before pointing in two or more heads and bursting. Most boils occur on hairy parts of the body or on areas of friction —

these include the armpits, the back of the neck, between the legs and buttocks, and in the nostrils. If left alone many boils will come to a head in about a week but some will take twice as long.

Mankind has been afflicted by boils for thousands of years. Some people are particularly prone to infections of this sort and find they recur whenever they are feeling particularly stressed or run down. Often the pain is so intense the sufferer can think of little else, and all sorts of treatments have been suggested to relieve the pain and bring the boil to a head more quickly.

One traditional method has been to lance the boil in order to allow the pus to escape. This is extremely painful for the patient and can often cause the infection to spread. Doctors today generally lance a boil only as a last resort and are more likely to advise rest to allow the body's natural defences to work, as well as applying a hot poultice to bring the boil to a head more quickly. They generally advise against the use of antiseptic creams or any other substance applied to the surface of the boil because these do not usually pass through the skin to the infection beneath.

This is where tea tree oil is different from other antiseptics. It has been shown to actually penetrate through the skin so that it can act on the bacteria beneath the surface. In addition, the oil actually breaks up the pus as a solvent. This unique action makes it an excellent treatment for boils. It is also unusually gentle, unlike many disinfectants, and will not irritate healthy tissue.

Once a boil bursts it is very important to stop the infection spreading to other parts of the body or to other people in the household. The affected part should be bathed regularly in a good antiseptic —

tea tree oil is excellent — and all clothes, sheets and towels should be washed in hot water and disinfectant. Something should also be added to the bathwater to kill the germs. Tea tree oil can be used very effectively for all these purposes.

There is an enormous amount of anecdotal evidence concerning the value of tea tree oil in the treatment of boils. An American doctor, Henry M. Feinblatt, M.D., F.A.C.P., from Brooklyn New York, conducted a controlled series of clinical studies to try to scientifically validate the evidence for the effectiveness of tea tree oil. He presented his results in a paper titled 'Cajeput-Type Oil for the Treatment of Furunculosis', which was published in the *Journal of the National Medical Association* in January 1960.

Feinblatt used as his subjects 35 patients who had come to his surgery complaining of furunculosis (boils), of which three were complicated by carbuncles. Twenty-five of the patients were treated with oil from the Australian plant *Melaleuca alternifolia* and the other ten were not. The method of application was that of painting the surface of the boil freely with the oil two or three times a day, after thoroughly cleaning the site.

The results showed that of the ten untreated control patients, five eventually needed to have their boils incised and in the other five cases, the infected site of the boil was still apparent after eight days. In the other twenty-five cases which had been treated with tea tree oil only one boil required incision. The infected site of the boil was removed completely in eight days in fifteen cases, while in six cases the boil, though still present, was reduced more than one half. In the other three cases the infected site was reduced by less than one half. There were no toxic effects of the treatment in any case, and only three of the patients complained of slight temporary stinging.

Feinblatt concluded that the oil of *Melaleuca alternifolia* 'encouraged more rapid healing without scarring than conservative treatment in the control series'. He felt that the high germicidal activity of the oil against *Staphylococcus aureus* accounted for the rapid improvement in the boils which were treated with it, and recommended tea tree oil should always be tried before surgical intervention.

Some medical practitioners have also reported successful treatment of boils using Melasol, which is an emulsion containing a 40 per cent solution of tea tree oil in a castor oil soap and containing about 13 per cent isopropyl alcohol. For a very severe boil, a gauze pad can be soaked in tea tree oil and placed over the boil for up to twelve hours. However, in most cases it is sufficient to apply the oil directly to the boil three times a day.

Bruises

A BRUISE IS the outward sign of bleeding beneath the skin as a result of pressure or a blow. Blood from damaged vessels seeps into the tissues causing swelling, discolouration and soreness. The characteristic changes in colour of bruised tissue are the result of the gradual degeneration of the components of the blood. A valuable first-aid treatment is to apply a cold compress to the area as soon as possible. Some people have also reported that tea tree oil dabbed directly onto the bruise will hasten the healing of the damaged tissue. Tea tree oil is able to penetrate through unbroken skin, deep into the tissue beneath it. It will also increase the blood-flow in the capillaries, so encouraging the rich healing blood to come to the aid of the damaged tissue with extra resources of oxygen and nutrients.

Burns and Sunburn

BURNS CAN BE among the most serious of common accidents as they carry associated risks of shock and infection. The dangers for very young children are especially serious because even a fairly small burn affects a proportionally larger area of the body.

The best immediate first-aid is to plunge the burnt area into cold water either from a running tap or into a bath — and leave it there for at least ten minutes or until the pain subsides. Burnt clothing which has stuck to the skin should not be removed, nor should any sticky ointments be smeared onto the injury. If the burn is serious or covers a large area of the body medical attention should be sought immediately.

Even a minor burn can be extremely painful and, if the skin is broken, may become infected. Tea tree oil has a mild anaesthetic effect and is particularly soothing for burns and inflamed skin. It also has well known antiseptic qualities which will greatly reduce any risk of infection. The oil can be applied directly to the burn or, if preferred, it can be used in the form of a non-greasy antiseptic cream.

There are numerous anecdotal accounts extolling the virtues of tea tree oil. One woman on a camping holiday bent down to pick up a glass beer bottle which she felt was dangerously close to the fire. As she grasped the bottle firmly she realised too late that it was red hot! Her fingers and palm were burned excruciatingly and she immediately plunged her painful hand into the cooling waters of a nearby creek. After half an hour the pain had not subsided so she and her family continued with their hike. When at last they finally arrived back at their tent (almost three hours later) the hand was still very painful so she went straight to the first-aid box, took out her bottle of tea tree oil — something they never leave home without — and sprinkled it liberally over her fingers. To her enormous relief, the pain subsided immediately and she was able to get on with preparing dinner for her family.

Now that such a wide range of effective sunscreens is available and people are becoming increasingly aware of the danger of over-exposure to the sun, there is really no excuse for allowing yourself to get sunburnt. However each summer there are some people who forget their sunburn cream or underestimate the length of time they have been lying on the beach. By the end of the day their skin is bright red and feels as though it has been stretched tightly across their shoulders. Every movement causes agonising pain and in many cases the skin will soon blister and then peel away, leaving an unsightly speckled back.

A cool bath or shower (with only a gentle spray) will bring some temporary relief. Then the skin should be gently coated with tea tree antiseptic cream or, in very severe cases, with pure tea tree oil. This will take the pain away almost instantly and will also help to stop blistering. It can be repeated as often as necessary. The relief is wonderful.

Cuts and Abrasions

IN MANY HOUSEHOLDS, particularly where there are young children, the most common injuries are slight cuts and grazes. Often these need little or no treatment except thorough cleaning to prevent any possible infection, so every family needs a bottle of disinfectant in the first-aid kit. Unfortunately, many of these disinfectants sting so much that the pain of the treatment is worse than the injury itself.

Tea tree oil has excellent antiseptic qualities — it has been shown to kill harmful bacteria even when diluted down to one part in a hundred. And yet it is so gentle in its action it will not sting the exposed raw skin, and even has mild anaesthetic quality. The oil can be applied directly from the bottle in its pure form or diluted into a soothing antiseptic cream.

E. Morris Humphery wrote in his article in the *Medical Journal of Australia* (vol. 1, 1930):

'Dirty wounds, such as are frequently seen as the result of street accidents, may be washed or syringed out with a 10% water solution, the solvent properties will loosen and the tissues will remain fresh and retain their natural colour. Dressings dipped in a 2.5% solution may then be applied, changed every 24 hours and healing will readily take place.'

One of the remarkable things about tea tree oil is that it actually appears to work better in an organic medium where pus or dirt are present, or deep inside the tissue. This is quite unusual as many common antiseptics are often rendered useless (and some even harm the skin) in the presence of organic debris. Tea tree oil has been found to work better on the skin or in pus-laden areas than it does in a test tube. It also acts to increase the blood flow in the capillaries, so encouraging this rich healing blood to come to the aid of the damaged skin with extra resources of oxygen, nutrients and germ-fighting white corpuscles.

Cystitis

THIS INFECTION OF the bladder is caused by a germ from the bowel entering the urethra and reaching the bladder. Because the urethra in females is shorter and closer to the anus, the condition is more common in women than in men. Symptoms include frequency of passing urine, cloudy urine sometimes with a 'fishy' smell, and also pain in the genitals when urine is passed. There may also be some fever. Usually the complaint lasts about four or five days, during which time patients are told to rest and drink as much fluid as possible. Sometimes antibiotics are prescribed, particularly if the condition becomes chronic or if attacks occur frequently.

Dr Paul Belaiche conducted a very interesting study on twenty-six patients, all of whom suffered from chronic cystitis and had been on courses of antibiotics without any definite success. Thirteen women were given tea tree oil orally — 24 mgs a day (to be swallowed in three doses of 8 mgs half an hour before meals). The other thirteen were given a placebo which smelled like tea tree oil.

Patients were examined after one month, three months and six months. The results were not spectacular and many of the patients in both groups needed to take short courses of antibiotics at the same time for severe attacks. However, after six months, seven of the patients who had been taking tea tree oil were cured of their symptoms while none of the control group showed any significant improvement. Belaiche concluded:

'From this first clinical approach it is apparent that the essential oil of *Melaleuca alternifolia* is effectively efficient for the treatment of chronic *colibacilli* cystitis. The absence of toxicity, the low level of irritation on the mucous membrane, its perfect general tolerance, and its high germicidal power . . . has convinced us that we are in possession of a MAJOR NEW ANTISEPTIC ESSENTIAL OIL FOR AROMATHERAPY.'

Dennis Stewart, a well known herbal practitioner and the Director of the Southern Cross Herbal College of New South Wales, is equally impressed by the healing qualities of tea tree oil. He writes: 'We use tea tree oil for urogenitary infections, particularly for vaginitis, cystitis, urethritis and fungal infections generally. The preparation is the preparation of choice in the primary treatment of these conditions. The preparation is used both orally and as a topical application, following the British Pharmacopoeia.'

Dental Care

THE VALUE OF tea tree oil in curing and preventing a variety of dental diseases has been recognised since the 1930s when an article in *The Australian Journal of Dentistry* (Aug. 1, 1930) deplored the use by some dentists of powerful antiseptic drugs to treat pockets of pus in the gums. While these often achieved the desired result they also destroyed surrounding healthy tissue and lowered the body's natural defences, leaving the mouth more vulnerable to the next crop of bacteria. The article pointed out that tea tree oil, while is was a very strong antiseptic (11–13 times stronger than carbolic) was also non-toxic and did not damage healthy tissue.

The most common dental diseases, which affect most people at some time, are dental decay and gingivitis. Dental decay begins with the formation of a stickly film called plaque on the teeth and gums. If this is not removed thoroughly it can form an acid which eats into the enamel of the tooth and begins the formation of dental caries.

Many people have found that tea tree oil helps to keep their teeth clean, as Sue Coffey of Lane Cove, New South Wales, wrote:

 'My dentist asked me if I had had my teeth cleaned by another dentist as I had no plaque and yet it was twelve months since my teeth had been cleaned. I put it down to rinsing my mouth daily with Ballinas (water miscible tea tree oil). It gives me a really healthy mouth and fresh breath, I love it.'

Other people have written praising the fresh taste (which can help to eliminate bad breath) and also the fact that their teeth look whiter.

Gingivitis affects nine out of ten people to some extent. It is an inflammation of the gums caused mainly by poor dental hygiene which leads to swelling and bleeding and, if untreated, may cause the teeth to become loose and eventually fall out. It is caused mainly by accumulation of plaque in the area where the tooth meets the gum. If ignored, gingivitis can develop into periodontitis, an inflammation of the structures supporting the teeth. Pockets of pus may accumulate around the teeth and serious ulcers form inside the mouth.

The best way to avoid gingivitis is by careful cleaning of the teeth, removal of plaque, and use of an antibacterial mouthwash. Tea tree oil has been shown to be extremely effective. It can be dabbed directly onto the gums or used as a mouthwash made from three drops of tea tree oil added to one third of a glass of water. The praise from numerous satisfied customers has been supported by reports from a number of registered dental practitioners. One wrote:

> 'In a 5% solution Melasol (tea tree oil) has helped considerably in cleaning up the mouth. After scaling the teeth Melasol used in an atomiser and sprayed rather forcibly between the interstitial spaces has greatly benefited the mouth. I have cleared up very quickly several cases of gingivitis with Melasol'.

Others have reported the use of tea tree oil for cleaning dental cavities, for cleaning septic canals, as a preparation for nerve capping, and to prevent infection after extractions or other dental operations.

In 1987 Dr L.J. Walsh of the Department of Social and Preventive Dentistry in the University of Queensland, and his colleague Dr J. Longstaff, a microbiologist, having read reports of the use of Oil of Melaleuca in medicine and dentistry because of its high germicidal activity and low toxicity to the patient, conducted a study to determine the effectiveness of tea tree oil against a wide variety of oral and non-oral pathogens. They used Broth and Agar dilution tests and found Oil of Melaleuca possessed considerable anti-microbial properties, especially against anaerobic and microaerophillic organisms and inhibited the growth of a number of organisms which are thought to play key roles in causing adult periodontitis.

Dermatitis

THIS IS A general term used to describe a number of skin disorders, many of which are allergies. Very often dermatitis is the result of skin hypersensitivity to certain irritants such as household cleansers, nylon, wool, metal, lubricating oil and cement. Nappy rash is an example of dermatitis caused by the ammonia in urine.

Symptoms of allergic dermatitis vary considerably but usually include inflammation, swelling, raised spots and itching. The most natural reaction of the sufferer from dermatitis is to scratch — this aggravates the condition and may also cause infection. Sometimes it is difficult to determine exactly what is causing dermatitis because the allergic reaction may occur some time after the initial contact. Some workers in industry have been handling particular substances for many years when suddenly, for no apparent reason, they develop an allergic reaction. In the same way, a particular brand of deodorant or after-shave which has been used for a long time may suddenly produce an allergic reaction.

Dermatitis is often very difficult to cure because it is necessary first to find the cause and then remove it. The usual treatment is with a soothing cream made of coal tar and a steroid cream to reduce the inflammation. When the skin has become infected antibiotic creams are sometimes prescribed as well.

There is a considerable amount of evidence from satisfied patients to show that tea tree oil is particularly effective in the treatment of dermatitis and other itching skin disorders (such as chicken pox). A most dramatic story comes from E. MacNamara, a resident of Sydney. She wrote this letter to the distributors of tea tree oil, Thursday Plantation:

'My husband, Mr MacNamara, contracted a severe cement dust allergy as a result of his industrial occupation and had been undergoing treatment for this for the past four years. The condition continued to deteriorate to the point where he was confined to a wheelchair because the skin of his feet and calves was so tender that contact with soft carpet, shoes or even bed clothes caused bleeding and great pain.

We tried hundreds of medicines prescribed by specialists and in fact our compensation records showed that we spent over $3000 in two years looking for a suitable cream. Finally, our doctor advised that it was most likely that amputation of both legs below the knee would be necessary within twelve months. I then saw a story on television about tea tree oil and decided it was worth trying. I purchased a bottle from my health food shop and we rubbed it all over the affected area. Within two weeks the condition had cleared up totally and now eleven months later there has been no recurrence whatsoever.'

Fungal Infections

A FUNGUS IS a simple form of plant life that forms a system of thin filaments called a mycelium. There is a wide variety of fungi and many of them, such as moulds, mushrooms and yeasts, are beneficial to man. Others live on humans as parasites and cause infections such as tinea and candidiasis (candida).

Since the discovery of antibiotics the incidence of fungal infections has actually increased. This is probably because the antibiotics destroy bacteria — the main biological competitors of fungi — thus increasing the chances of infection.

Tea tree oil has been shown to be an extremely effective treatment for a wide variety of fungal infections, often bringing about a cure when all other treatments have failed.

Tinea (Athlete's Foot)
Medically known as *Tinea pedis*, this condition is a form of ringworm. The tinea fungi can attack any area of the skin but the damp, warm parts of the body are most vulnerable. *Tinea cruris* affects the groin, *Tinea capitis* affects the scalp, and *Tinea barbae*, sometimes known as barber's rash, affects the beard. The most common form is *Tinea pedis*, commonly known as athlete's foot. This attacks the warm moist area between the toes and on the soles and sides of the feet. The skin between the toes becomes soggy, flaking and peeling, and small blisters and rashes occur around the toes and soles. Sometimes the soles and heels may become covered with white scales and the underlying skin is bright red with inflammation.

Tinea is highly infectious and spreads rapidly through communities such as schools where people use the same showers and may share towels. It is aggravated by wearing synthetic socks and shoes which do not allow the feet to 'breathe'.

Tea tree oil has been successfully applied to a

number of fungal infections and is particularly good
for tinea. As early as 1937, A.R. Penfold reported
the use of tea tree oil to cure many foot problems
and cited the example of the Surgeon Lieutenant of
H.M.S. Sussex, stationed at Alexandria in Egypt,
who cured an outbreak of tinea among the ship's
company by regular applications of Ti-trol (pure tea
tree oil).

In 1972 Moreton Walker conducted a very thorough study on the use of tea tree oil for several foot
problems including tinea. He presented his results in
an award winning paper titled 'Clinical Investigation
of Australian *Melaleuca Alternifolia* Oil for a Variety of Common Foot Problems'. Walker had first
used tea tree oil years earlier when it had been recommended to him as a super-potent fungicide and
germicide. Since then he had used it on a large
number of patients and had been very impressed by
the results.

Walker used the oil in three different preparations; firstly as pure tea tree oil, secondly as Melasol
(a solution containing 40 per cent oil of *Melaleuca
alternifolia* and 13 per cent isopropyl alcohol in a
special emulsion which mixes with water in any pro-
portion) and thirdly as Australian Tea Tree Ointment (an emollient ointment preparation containing
lanolin and chlorophyl along with 8 per cent tea tree
oil). All these products were supplied by the Meta-
bolic Products Corporation in the United States.

Sixty patients were involved in the study. Eight of
these had been told to use the pure tea tree oil, forty
to use the solution Melasol and twenty the ointment.
The study took place over a period of six years and
treatment times varied from three weeks to four
years. At the end of that time fifty-eight of the pa-

tients had found significant relief. For thirty-eight of the subjects the problem had been completely cured while for many others the symptoms had disappeared but laboratory examination of samples of the patients' skin showed that the organism still remained in their bodies.

It is interesting to note that tea tree oil seems to work on tinea just as well when it is diluted. Walker concluded that 'the various dilutions of Australian *Melaleuca alternifolia* oil eradicates or improves the symptoms of *Tinea pedis* with continuous daily use by the patient at home.'

A simple home remedy for tinea is to wash and dry the affected area thoroughly, then apply pure tea tree oil twice a day. If no improvement occurs within seven days medical advice should be sought.

Other Foot Problems
Many of the patients in Walker's study were suffering from complaints other than tinea and some of these responded very well to his treatment. In fact, Walker thought the most important information brought to light by his study was that 'the unpleasant and embarrassing bromidrotic condition responds quickly and rather permanently to *Melaleuca alternifolia*'. Bromidrosis is the medical term for 'smelly feet' and is caused by malodorous perspiration. Most patients found that rubbing their feet daily with the 40 per cent solution of tea tree oil left their feet sweet smelling all day. Some people, meanwhile, prefer to add five to ten drops of pure tea tree oil to warm water and soak their feet in this for five minutes each night.

Some of Walker's patients were given the 40 per cent solution of tea tree oil to use on corns, bunions,

painful hammer toes, deep seated calluses and cracks
and fissures around the thickened skin of the heel.
All reported significant improvement and in many
cases the problem disappeared. Indeed, 96.4 per cent
of Walker's subjects improved when using tea tree
oil on their foot problems.

Paronychia
This fungal infection, which develops under the
fingernails or toenails, has also been shown to respond very well to tea tree oil. It is a notoriously difficult condition to cure. The cuticle becomes red and
painful with a slight discharge, and if the condition
persists the nail becomes ridged and furrowed and
often there is discolouration below the nail. The nail
becomes quite distorted and eventually may have to
be removed.

Several doctors have written recommending the
use of tea tree oil for this condition but none has
summed up the results quite so well as Mr John Pike
from Collaroy Plateau, New South Wales, who
wrote to the suppliers of Ballinas (tea tree oil) to
congratulate them on their product. He wrote:

'For eight years my wife has had a nasty fungal
infection in her fingernails and not one specialist
could fix it. A friend suggested she try Ballinas oil
and it's hard to believe in two days the improvement started. After three weeks the nails had grown
out and have been perfect ever since. You should ad-
vertise this is a medical journal.'

Dr Paul Belaiche, Professor of Phytotherapy at
the Faculty of Medicine in the University of Paris
Nord, treated eleven patients with nail bed infections
by applying tea tree oil twice a day for one to three

months. Eight of them recovered completely.

To treat paronychia at home, the infected nail should be soaked in tea tree oil for five minutes and massaged well twice a day for up to two weeks. If there is no improvement after this time the treatment should be discontinued.

Ringworm

This contagious fungus is also known medically as tinea. It is a result of the same fungus that causes athlete's foot (*Tinea pedis*) and can be caught from other people, from animals (especially dogs and cats) and from the soil. The name 'ringworm' is misleading because there is no worm involved, but the infection forms a ring because the inflamed patches extend at their edges while their centres return to a normal skin appearance. It can occur on any parts of the body and, if left untreated, may persist for months or even years. When it occurs on the scalp (*Tinea capitis*) it causes the hairs to break off in each patch of infection and in severe cases may give the hair a moth-eaten appearance.

Ringworm can be treated very effectively with tea tree oil and usually takes only a few days to disappear. The affected parts should be carefully washed and dried and then tea tree oil applied twice a day. Combs, hairbrushes, sheets and towels and all clothing which has come into contact with the infection should be washed in a solution of tea tree oil — this is much more effective than ordinary antiseptic.

Dhobi Itch

This condition, also known as *Tinea cruris*, is a very common type ringworm which affects the groin, usually in men. Inflamed pimples develop on the inside of the upper thigh and soon merge to form a scaly red patch with a distinct edge. It causes very troublesome itching and can be quite embarrassing. The best treatment is to wash and dry the area thoroughly and apply tea tree oil twice a day. Tight, synthetic clothing can aggravate the condition and should be avoided, especially in summer when the weather is often hot and humid.

Candidiasis (also known as Thrush or Moniliasis)

Today more and more people are becoming aware of this infection caused by the yeast-like fungus *Candida albicans*. There is some evidence that its incidence is actually increasing because of the use of antibiotics and corticosteroid drugs to treat other conditions. These drugs can cause chemical changes in the body that destroy the body's immunity to candidiasis and encourage the fungus to grow.

It is generally recognised that some people are more prone to thrush than others. These include overweight people with deep skin clefts, babies, diabetics, people who are generally debilitated or who are taking steroid or antibiotic drugs, and women whose hormone levels have been altered as a result of pregnancy or the use of oral contraceptives.

Candida albicans mostly affects the warm, moist parts of the body such as the folds of the skin, the genitals, the buttocks and under the breasts. In women the most common site of the infection is in the vagina, where symptoms include itching and inflammation and a thick, milky white discharge. Although an attack may only last a few days, it will usually recur. In babies, nappy rash may be due to thrush or they may contract candidiasis of the mouth while passing along the vagina during the birth. If thrush is sexually transmitted from a woman to her partner it causes balanitis, an inflammation of the end of the penis. Paronychia, a chronic infection of the fingernails often found in people whose hands are frequently in hot water, is also caused by the fungus *Candida albicans*, and so are some painful cracks around the angles of the mouth.

Because candidiasis is infectious, it seems logical to treat it with an antiseptic. However, this can often aggravate the problem because antiseptics will often irritate already sensitive skin and cause the condition to worsen. This is the tremendous advantage of tea tree oil. It has been shown to be an extremely powerful anti-fungal treatment yet, because of its low cineol content, it is very gentle used in the correct dilutions and will not irritate even the most delicate skin such as that around the genitals.

In 1985 Dr Paul Belaiche carried out a study to determine the effectiveness of tea tree oil in treating vaginal infections of *Candida albicans*. Belaiche had been impressed for some time with the antibacterial properties of various essential oils, such as the Cinammon of Ceylon and China, Spanish Oregano and the Savory of Provence, but had found they were all 'aggressively irritating to the vaginal mucous membranes'. On the other hand, he had noticed that the oil of *Melaleuca alternifolia*, while it had a 'remarkable anti-fungal action', could also be used for as long as two months without causing any irritation of the mucous membrane.

With these two factors in mind, he began a systematic study of the treatment of twenty-eight young women (average age thirty-four) suffering from vaginal infections of *Candida albicans*. He used essential oil of *Melaleuca alternifolia* with the following characteristics:

specific gravity = 0.8999
optical rotation = +9 degrees
refractive index = 1.4750

The principal contituents of his oil were:
cineole 1,8   9.1%
p-cymene   16.4%
terpinen-4-ol   31%
alphaterpineol   3.5%

The patients were instructed to insert a specially prepared capsule into the vagina each night before retiring and to use some sort of protection to absorb the nocturnal vaginal emissions. The capsules were oval in shape, weighing 2 grams and manufactured from pre-cut gelatin sheets; each contained 2 centigrams of essential oil of *Melaleuca alternifolia.* Vaginal insertion was felt to be particularly effective as the oil acted directly on the fungus and was also absorbed directly into the blood vessels of the pelvic area, so bypassing the hepatic filter.

Of the twenty-eight patients only one felt vaginal burning and she stopped treatment. After thirty days twenty-three patients were completely cured and the burning white discharge (leucorrhea) had ceased. Four patients had to continue treatment for a longer period but they did show some improvement. Belaiche concluded: 'The essential oil of Melaleuca has entered the team of major essential oils and emerges as an antiseptic and anti-fungal weapon of the first order in phyto-aromatherapy.'

Belaiche's findings have been supported by a number of medical practitioners. Many prefer to administer treatment by saturating a tampon in tea tree oil. This is a routine method used at the Annandale Women's Centre in Sydney. The oil can also be diluted in the ratio of 5 mls tea tree oil to 500 mls water, and used as a douche.

Many naturopaths believe that *Candida albicans* can be controlled by eliminating from the diet those foods which cause it to thrive. Unfortunately this can lead to a very restrictive diet. A leading Sydney naturopath, Karin Cutter, believes the special diet should be supplemented by the use of an anti-fungal agent and warns that not all strains of Candida respond to every anti-fungal agent. She quotes the case of Baby Sarah, a tiny patient only a few months old, who suffered from projectile vomiting. She had undergone exhaustive medical tests but no cause could be found. The baby's diet was changed to fresh, raw goat's milk with small amounts of lactobacilli, and Karin suggested the parents should add two drops of tea tree oil into her bath water as an anti-yeast agent. The vomiting ceased very quickly and two months later Sarah was still thriving and gaining weight steadily.

Karin Cutter believes *Melaleuca alternifolia*'s value in the fight against yeast infections 'is clearly inestimable'. She suggests all Candida sufferers will benefit greatly from adding a teaspoon of this oil to their bathwater, inhaling the vapours of five drops in a bowl of hot water at least once a week, and gargling with a solution of three drops in warm water. However, she does warn her patients to be sure to buy their tea tree oil from a reputable manufacturer so that they can be sure that the highly toxic cineol content is well below the guidelines set by the Health Department.

Hair Care

THE GENTLE ACTION of tea tree oil on the skin and its excellent antiseptic qualities make it a suitable ingredient for hair care preparations. Some users of tea tree oil who have been accustomed to adding it to their bathwater have mixed a few drops into their own shampoo with excellent results. Thursday Plantation is now marketing two shampoos — one for normal to oily hair and the other for dry hair. The shampoos have a fresh, clean smelling fragrance and are prepared from a blend of 2 per cent tea tree oil with sodium lauryl ether sulphate, citric acid, sodium chloride, coconut diethanolamide and water.

The tea tree oil acts on any bacterial or fungal infections of the scalp and has remarkable solvent properties which help to clear blocked pores and clogged hair follicles, thereby allowing the natural body oils to flow more freely and provide the natural conditioning which leaves hair healthy and manageable. Tea tree oil conditioner is also available for use after the shampoo.

As early as 1939, Robert Goldsborough, a chemist working in soap perfumery and cosmetics, reported the use of a liquid shampoo containing 3 per cent tea tree oil as a treatment for dandruff. The results were excellent and he anticipated a good market for such a product.

Tea tree oil shampoo is an excellent treatment for the unsightly cradle cap which so often coats the heads of tiny babies. Five drops of tea tree oil should be mixed with olive oil and rubbed gently into the scalp. After five minutes the baby's hair should be washed with tea tree oil shampoo and then rinsed with clear water.

Head lice, (nits, pediculosis)
Every school suffers from periodic outbreaks of infestation of these tiny insects which suck blood from the skin (usually on the scalp) and leave it feeling very itchy. The eggs (called nits) are small, greyish white dots which adhere firmly to the hair and are very difficult to remove. They can be seen quite clearly when the hair is parted or lifted at the back and examined closely. Head lice pass very quickly from one child to another and will attack even the cleanest heads. They are often treated by washing the hair with a special shampoo containing the chemical gamma benzine hexachloride. Those people who would prefer not to expose their children to too many chemicals might prefer to use tea tree oil shampoo boosted with ten drops of pure tea tree oil. The shampoo should be left on for ten minutes then rinsed and the treatment repeated after one week. Care should be taken not to let this mixture get into the eyes. Tea tree oil is a natural oil with strong antiseptic qualities and is an effective insecticide. This treatment also leaves the hair in beautiful condition.

Herpes

THIS IS THE family name for a large group of viruses, the best known of which are probably cold sores, genital herpes and shingles.

A cold sore is an inflamed, blister-like sore which occurs mostly on the lips or face and lasts about a week. Some people are particularly prone to cold sores and find they recur whenever they are overtired or stressed, when they have some other infection such as a cold or 'flu, or even when they are exposed to extreme sunlight or cold winds. Cold sores are infectious and can be spread to other parts of the body or to other people. They do not respond to antibiotics and there is no known medical cure, so treatment usually involves merely soothing the pain and trying to stop further infections.

Unfortunately many antiseptics are too harsh and merely cause further irritation to already sensitive skin. However, tea tree oil can be applied directly to the lesions without causing pain and its strong antiseptic action helps to clear up the infection more quickly and stops it from spreading. It is very easy to administer — simply dab it on straight from the bottle — and is particularly effective if used when the cold sore first starts to develop.

News of the merits of tea tree oil is most often spread by word of mouth, as shown by this letter from Roger McDonald of Surfers Paradise, Queensland:

'I suffered with cold sores caused by sunburn and my skin specialist told me there was no cure, as it is a virus. My neighbour suggested Ballinas (tea tree oil) and to my surprise it really works. My specialist doctor now recommends your oil for cold sore blisters.'

A more distressing and increasingly common complaint is genital herpes. This is a sexually transmitted disease which is increasing at an alarming rate.

It is characterised by itching and reddened skin on the genital areas which soon erupts into small painful ulcers. The first attack is usually the worst: the blisters are extremely painful and may last two or three weeks and be accompanied by a general feeling of malaise. After this, recurrent attacks will occur — often precipitated by stress, other infections, or even sexual activity. These tend to be milder and only last four or five days, but they are still very troublesome.

Genital herpes is an extremely contagious disease and is transmitted by sexual activity, so patients are advised to refrain from sex for at least a week after an attack. It is generally more severe in women and there is the additional complication that a pregnant woman may pass the herpes virus on to her unborn child.

Like cold sores, genital herpes does not respond to antibiotics and there is no known cure. The best that can be hoped for is to relieve the pain and itching and stop the spread of infection. Several sufferers have found that dabbing tea tree oil on the blisters seems to promote healing and stop the development of new sores. It is one of the few antiseptics which can be used without causing excruciating pain to the delicate sexual organs. Some people also find it helpful to add tea tree oil to the bath water (thirty drops is suggested) or even to make a diluted mixture and use it in a pump spray.

As tea tree oil works so well with cold sores and genital herpes, it is likely it would also work in relieving shingles. This extremely painful condition (also called *Herpes zoster*) which often affects elderly people, is at present treated only with analgesics. Attacks can be cut short if the condition is diagnosed very early and anti-viral 'paint' applied to the spots. As tea tree oil has no harmful side-effects it could be very useful to apply it to any red spots along the intercostal nerves under the ribs, as this is where shingles generally develop.

Insect Bites

THE WARM AUSTRALIAN weather and our love of the great outdoors leave most Australians particularly vulnerable to an enormous variety of bites and stings. Every new arrival to the country is warned of the dangers of spiders and insects and every household is equipped with a number of commercial products designed to repel these creatures or, if this is not possible, to relieve the pain and itchiness of their stings. Unfortunately some of these products contain such harmful chemicals that many people would prefer to put up with the insects!

This is no longer necessary. As some people have known for a long time, tea tree oil makes an excellent natural insect repellent and can also be dabbed directly onto bites to take away some of the itchiness and to prevent the infection which sometimes results when people, especially small children, scratch their bites until they bleed. What is more, because it is so mild in its action, tea tree oil can be used over and over again on the same area with little fear of causing irritation to the skin.

The early tea tree cutters were among the first to discover the repellent properties of tea tree oil. They applied it to their socks to ward off the leeches which abounded in the tea trees' native habitat. The oil can also be used to remove leeches which have already attached themselves to the skin. It should be applied directly to the leech and the surrounding skin. The leech will drop off immediately and the bite will be treated against infection. The same treatment can be used for ticks and once the tick is dead it can be easily removed.

Many people dab tea tree oil onto their exposed

skin to protect it from mosquito, sandfly and flea bites. Some prefer to mix it with a little baby oil to make a lotion which can be spread more easily. For stings from insects like bees and wasps, where the pain can persist for some time, tea tree oil has been found to give fast relief.

For pets who are plagued by summertime itching from those tiny black fleas which are so hard to eradicate from even the cleanest household, Thursday Plantation has developed a special anti-itch shampoo. This can be used as often as necessary and has the double benefit of soothing the animal's reddened and inflamed skin and also destroying the insects. For extra protection between shampoos the fur can be wiped with a moist sponge sprinkled with ten to twenty drops of pure tea tree oil.

One amazing story was sent to Thursday Plantation by Mr Harry Henry Bungwahl of Taree, New South Wales. He wrote:

'A rather extraordinary episode happened to me recently involving your tea tree oil. I was bitten by a funnel-web spider . . . It happened at night time about 1 a.m. He gave me a vicious bite, in fact it was very painful . . . I lay down on the bed and tried to think of some way to soothe the pain of the bite, which was very severe. I then thought of the small bottle of tea tree oil that was in the bathroom. My wife went and got it and applied some to the bite and there was an immediate easing of the pain . . . My wife then went to ring up Taree Hospital, and while she was doing that, I gave a further application of tea tree oil to the bite and the bite in a short time stopped being painful! My son drove me to the Taree Hospital — the foot was no longer painful but my lips and fingers were still tingling.

The spider was identified as a male funnel-web spider all right. I was given no treatment but was kept under observation for a period of four hours, and then discharged . . . The tea tree oil definitely checked the pain of the bite.'

The bite of a funnel-web can be fatal, particularly for small children, and since after many years of research an effective antidote has been developed, anyone with a suspected funnel-web bite should go straight to the nearest hospital. However, as tea tree oil does no damage it would certainly do no harm to apply some while waiting for medical attention, and it may even do some good. In an isolated situation, far from medical assistance, a bottle of tea tree oil could literally be a life-saver.

Muscular Aches and Pains

MOST PEOPLE TODAY would like to have a healthy and active body. However, the sedentary lifestyles of many workers do nothing to develop this, so those who want to increase their fitness need to engage in some sort of regular activity. This usually takes the form of some type of organised sport, aerobics or a work-out at the gym.

All of these activities can achieve their desired aim if performed regularly but unfortunately many people find they exercise only sporadically, when they have a burst of energy or when they feel guilty about their usual lethargic state. This sudden muscular exertion is likely to cause all sorts of muscular strain and often leaves the body feeling very stiff and sore.

A few drops of tea tree oil rubbed into the muscles before and immediately after strenuous sport can help to relieve these feelings. So too can a relaxing hot bath with 1 ml of tea tree oil added to the water.

Respiratory Tract Infections

COLDS, SORE THROATS and 'flu are the illnesses which affect most of us most frequently and yet they are notoriously difficult to cure. They are usually virus infections which do not respond to antibiotics. However, modern man has been conditioned to expect an instant cure for most complaints so chemist shops are full of a bewildering range of products to soothe the various symptoms of colds and 'flu. Many of these have only psychosomatic value and some contain substances which are potentially harmful, especially if used frequently.

One of the safest and most effective home remedies available (and also one of the cheapest) is a bottle of tea tree oil. For the child with a heavy cold who wakes up in the night complaining he 'can't breathe', a few drops of trea tree oil can be sprinkled on a tissue, or on the pillow, then held near the nose to provide almost instant relief. An alternative is to rub the oil directly on to the nose — it will usually not sting. It is very reassuring to know that the oil of *Melaleuca alternifolia* is harmless and you can repeat the treatment as often as necessary.

Some people prefer to mix tea tree oil with hot water and use it as an inhalant — this, too, provides excellent results. Five drops are sufficient for a bowl of hot water or the oil can be added to a vapouriser. Many people find the humid steamy conditions created by a vapouriser in a small closed room very helpful for soothing croup-like coughs and sinus congestion. Tea tree oil can also be rubbed into the chest and back or sprinkled onto the pillow at bedtime. Three drops of tea tree oil in a spoonful of honey can be sipped slowly to soothe a tickling cough.

The strong antiseptic qualities of tea tree oil make it very effective in treating sore throats, especially in the early stages. A gargle can be made from three to six drops of tea tree oil in a glass of warm water and used twice a day. Another method is to put three drops of tea tree oil into a spoonful of honey or a sugar cube and suck it slowly. Three drops of tea tree oil can also be added to a quarter of a glass of juice and sipped slowly (lemon juice is probably the best, as this will give a double benefit).

A bottle of tea tree oil is something no household should be without. It can be used to bring relief from a whole range of minor complaints and so save the expense of buying different proprietory products for specific symptoms. It is invaluable too for the travel-ler — the bottle is small and light and can be tucked into the corner of a bag where it will be easily avail-able when needed.

The feelings of people all over Australia who have discovered this amazingly versatile medicine have been summed up by Mrs Nolene Denize from Kambah, A.C.T., who wrote:

'Our family is using this oil as a general medicine-cupboard basic and so far I have noted its effectiveness as a gargle for sore throats, cure for tinea, general antiseptic and sting soother. I am very impressed.'

Vaginal Infections

INFLAMMATION OF THE vagina and vulva involving discharge, itching or soreness may arise from many different causes. One of these, thrush or candidiasis, has been discussed under the heading 'Fungal Infections'. Another common complaint *Trichomonas vaginitis*, is an infection caused by the parasitic protozoan *Trichomonas vaginalis*. It causes soreness of the vulva and an offensive yellowish discharge which may appear frothy. Vaginitis may also be caused by a bacterial infection, in which case there is an irritating whitish discharge.

Conventional treatment of all these complaints usually involves extra attention to hygiene but unfortunately frequent washing can actually aggravate the problem either by irritating already sensitive skin or by killing the lactobacilli — naturally occurring bacteria which form an essential part of the vagina's natural defence. Antibiotic drugs also have this effect, so should be avoided where possible. Some women use vaginal douches or deodorants but these, too, can often be harmful for the same reasons.

Fortunately a number of medical practitioners have found that tea tree oil can be used to clear up vaginal infections without having undesirable side effects.

In 1962 Eduardo F. Pena, a doctor from Miami, Florida, conducted a very useful study which was published in *Obstetrics and Gynaecology* (Vol. 19, no. 6, pp.793–795).

His paper was titled 'Melaleuca Alternifolia Oil: *its use for Trichomonal Vaginitis and other Vaginal Infections*'. Pena based his study on 130 women, 96 of them suffering from trichonomal vaginitis and the others from thrush and cervicitis. Pena considered most of the complaints had been caused by faulty menstrual hygiene associated with the use of unsanitary menstrual pads or tampons. He wanted to determine the value and safety of *Melaleuca alternifolia* oil for use as a vaginal douche and for topical application. He was also keen to observe any side-effects and determine the proper strength of the oil for safety and efficiency. Another group of fifty women were used as controls and were treated with standard anti-trichonomal suppositories. The tea tree oil was applied diluted, by means of saturated tampons and douches, but was not given orally.

All 130 patients were treated successfully and the results were similar to the control group. Many patients commented on the pleasant odour of the tea tree oil, its cooling, soothing effect and its efficiency in removing unpleasant vaginal odours. None complained of any irritation or burning. Pena concluded:

— 'Australian *Melaleuca alternifolia* oil in suitable dilutions was found to be highly effective in the treatment of trichonomal vaginitis, moniliasis, cervicitis and chronic endocervicitis.

— A 40 per cent solution of the oil produced no irritation, burning or other side-effects.

— A 20 per cent solution is effective for treating cervicitis.

— Daily vaginal douches with 0.4 per cent of the oil in one quart of water proved a safe and effective treatment of the vaginal infections under consideration.

— The clinical evidence supports the laboratory
tests which show that Australian *Melaleuca
alternifolia* oil is a penetrating germicide and
fugistat with the additional properties of dissolv-
ing pus and debris.'

It is important to remember that vaginal discharge
can be associated with other conditions such as dia-
betes so if it persists medical attention should be
sought.

For simple vaginal cleansing a douche can be
made of 5 mls pure tea tree oil with half a litre of
clean water and shaken together. This concentration
should produce only a slight tingling effect.

Varicose Ulcers

THESE OPEN SORES, which are usually painless,
may form on the lower leg when the veins are
not functioning properly, often as a result of varicose
veins. They frequently become infected and are often
very slow to heal.

In the early 1960s an American pamphlet titled
'Australian Tea Tree Oil' reported the successful
treatment of a varicose ulcer without the complete
rest that is usually necessary before healing can take
place. The wound was first bathed in a warm diluted
solution of tea tree oil, then covered with a pad
which had been saturated in a solution of three parts
olive oil to one part pure tea tree oil. It healed much
more rapidly than would otherwise have been
expected.

Warts

EVERYONE IS FAMILIAR with these small hard growths on the skin which, although harmless, are often so unsightly that most people want to remove them as quickly as possible. They are caused by a virus, are slightly contagious, and seem to affect children more than adults. If left alone, warts will eventually disappear but many people are not prepared to wait months or years for the wart to take its natural course. There is a huge range of recommended 'wart cures' ranging from the old practice of trying a string round a piece of raw meat and burying it at midnight, right through to burning off with electrically heated platinum needle. Some wart pastes and paints, while they do remove the horny skin of the wart, also cause considerable damage to the healthy skin around it.

Some people have found their warts disappear quite quickly if dabbed three times a day with tea tree oil. This remedy seems particularly effective for plantar warts which are deeply embedded in the soles of the feet and can be very painful to walk on.

5
New Findings

IN THE TWO YEARS since this book was first published some further significant developments have taken place in the Tea Tree Oil story.

In 1986 the Australian Tea Tree Industry Association (ATTIA) was founded with Christopher Dean as Chairman and some sixty members active within the Industry. This association has focused on the standardisation of Tea Tree Oil, on the progressive development of excellence within the industry and more recently on coordinating research and co-operation between members and appropriate Australian State and Federal Government authorities.

A two-day seminar at Byron Bay, northern New South Wales, in 1989 led to a substantial Joint Industry and Government Funded Research programme. This programme offers up to A$750,000 to be used over three years to develop agricultural, clinical and market skills for the Tea Tree Oil industry. The programme is administered jointly by ATTIA and the Rural Industries Research Development Corporation (RIRDC) in Canberra.

Research into areas as diverse as oil yield variables

and double blind clinical trials on fungal conditions (tinea) are sponsored by this excellent initiative.

In December 1990, a comprehensive clinical trial comparing the action of Tea Tree Oil with Benzoyl Peroxide in the treatment of acne was published by the Medical Journal of Australia under guidance from Professor Barneston, at the University of Sydney and Dr Phillip Altman, a specialist in pharmaceutical consultancy. Their study revealed the clear efficacy of Tea Tree Oil with an activity similar, if slightly slower than Benzoyl Peroxide preparation.

This paper confirms under scientific scrutiny, with a high standard of methodology, some of the results which have been observed repeatedly since the first medical trials were reported in the 1920s.

New Frontiers

AUSTRALIAN Tea Tree Oil has now commenced large scale production with major plantations such as Australian Plantations, Natural Extracts, Australian Tea Tree Estates and Melacare joining Thursday Plantation in the production and promotion of Tea Tree Oil worldwide. For the first time large quantities of good therapeutic grade oil, well researched, will be available for global use. Tea Tree Oil and related products are now available widely in the U.S.A. and Canadian health markets, in the U.K., Sweden, Finland, Holland, France, Italy, Israel, Malaysia, Singapore, Korea and New Zealand.

Around the world the same basic and constant first aid needs are found and the universal appeal of Tea Tree Oil is growing.

Bill Mollison, an Australian Ecologist, famous for developing the concept of Permaculture, reports how he regularly visits Rwanda in Central Africa. He always carries large quantities of Tea Tree Oil as it is so effective for the vast range of skin parasites which afflict residents of this poor tropical country. The oil is equally at home in jungles as in Manhattan skyscrapers, where many New York office workers keep it in the office desk drawer as a staple first aid kit.

Exciting new horizons for Tea Tree Oil are unfolding. Commonwealth Industrial Gases (C.I.G.), a major Australian corporation, has developed a treatment programme for air conditioning ducts in large buildings, using a "Bactigas" to create a "Healthizone" in the building. To explain: a controlled dose of Tea Tree Oil is misted through an air conditioning system on a regular basis to inhibit mould, fungi and bacteria which can thrive in the warm, moist, dark tunnels which duct the air through buildings. Better air to breathe, less respiratory infections, less mould on walls, less contamination of food processing areas etc., are all results proven to occur when this system operates.

Further exciting research is now underway to test Tea Tree Oil as a post harvest dip for stonefruit, strawberries, mangoes and other fruit – a non toxic and effective way to supplant existing poisonous treatments. So far the tests have been very encouraging.

Tea Tree Oil has many possible applications in agricultural use from delousing sheep to tick treatments, pest control and collar rot treatments for orchard trees.

Good results have been reported in treating fungi in carpets and also eradicating vermin such as cockroaches and fleas from houses.

All these applications require extensive research to establish full safety and efficacy. A fruitful line of research is currently underway at Macquarie University in Sydney where Professor Lyall Williams, assisted by Vicki Home, has started to compare and contrast the action of specific oil varieties against specific fungi, yeast and bacteria. The results so far indicate great precision and heightened activity levels are readily attainable in the products of the future.

Toxicity

ATTIA sponsored a comprehensive range of toxicity studies which have given a reasonable basis for professional users of Tea Tree Oil to prepare products with no chance of serious misuse. For casual users it is important to stress that Tea Tree Oil must not be indiscriminately taken internally as it, in common with all essential oils, has a significant toxicity sufficient to cause concern if quantities such as tablespoonsful (5ml) or more were to be ingested by young children.

Dog and cat owners are cautioned against using full strength concentrated Tea Tree Oil on their pets as this may be too strong for small animals. Reports (most anecdotal) indicate the oil may penetrate the spinal column and interfere with muscular co-ordination if too much is applied neat to a sensitive animal. Sensible doses are contained in professionally produced products which are excellent to use, with no possible risk to the animal.

New Findings on Acne

A RECENT scientifically controlled 'blind' trial was carried out to compare the effect of Tea Tree Oil against Benzoyl Peroxide — a widely used acne treatment. Tea Tree Oil, at 5%, compared favourably with the Benzoyl peroxide. Although a bit slower to act at first, the effects were quite comparable after a few weeks and with the great advantage that Tea Tree Oil caused much fewer harsh side effects than the caustic Benzoyl Peroxide preparation.

This study, involving 124 patients, was carried out by Professor Barnetson at Sydney University and published in the prestigious Medical Journal of Australia in October 1990. It offers conclusive proof of the efficacy and low toxicity of Tea Tree Oil. Observers have noted that, were the Tea Tree Oil product to be increased in strength, or applied more frequently, then the results may well indicate that Tea Tree Oil acts as fast, or faster than Benzoyl Peroxide; thus proving to be superior in every way.

Bibliography

Bassett, Pannowitz and Barnetson, 'A comparative study of tea-tree oil versus benzoylperoxide in the treatment of acne' *The Medical Journal of Australia*, October 1990. Vol. 153. pp.455–458.

Beer, Christopher, 'Australian Tea Tree Oil' *Nature and Health,* Vol.6, No. 3. Spring 1985. pp.3–6.

Belaiche, Dr Paul, 'L'Huile essentielle de Melaleuca alternifolia (Cheel) dans les infections urinaires colibacillaires chroniques idiopathiques.' *Phytotherapy,* September 1985. No. 15, Paris. 9–12.

Belaiche, Dr Paul, 'L'Huile essentielle de Melaleuca alternifolia (Cheel) dans les infections vaginales a candida albicans.' *Phytotherapy,* September 1985. No. 15, Paris. 13–14.

Belaiche, Dr Paul, 'L'Huile essentielle de Melaleuca alternifolia (Cheel) dans les infections cutanee's.' *Phytotherapy,* September 1985. No. 15, Paris. 15–18.

Beylier, M.F., 'Bacteriostatic Activity of Some Australian Essential Oils.' *Perfumer & Flavourist,* 4:23. April/May 1979. pp.23–25.

Coutts, M., 'The Bronchoscopic Treatment of Bronchiectasis,' *Medical Journal of Australia.* July, 1937.

Feinblatt, Henry M. 'Cajeput-Type Oil for the Treatment of Furunculosis'. *Journal of the National Medical Association,* vol.52:1. January 1960. pp.32–34.

Garnero, M.J., 'L'Huile essentielle de "Tea Tree" d'Australie. *Phytotherapy,* September 1985. No. 15, Paris.

Goldsborough, Robert E., 'Ti-Tree Oil', *Manufacturing Perfumer,* February 1939. pp.45, 58.

Goldsborough, Robert E., 'Ti-Tree Oil', *The Manufacturing Chemist*, February 1939. pp. 57, 58, 60.

Guenther, Ernest, 'Tea Tree Oils', *Soap and Sanitary Chemicals*, August/September 1942.

Guenther, Ernest, 'Australian Tea Tree Oils', *Perfumery and Essential Oil Record*, September 1968.

Guenther, E.S., 'Australian Tea Tree Oils; Report of a Field Survey', *Perfumes and Essences Organizational Report*, September 1986.

Guenther, E., *The Essential Oils*, Vol.IV.

Holland, E.H., 'Results of a series of investigations carried out on the Germicidal, Disinfectant and Bacteriostatic action of Melasol (*Melaleuca alternifolia*).' unpublished paper, Sydney University, 1941.

Lassak, E., *Australian Medical Plants*. Methuen, Sydney, 1984.

Laakso, P.V., 'Fractionation of Tea Tree Oil (*Melaleuca alternifolio*).' *Scientiae Pharmeceuticae*, 25:485, 1966.

Low, D., Rowal B.D., & Griffin, W.J., 'Antibacterial Action of the Essential Oils of Some Australian Myrtaceae.' *Planta Medica*, 26:184, 1974.

Miller, Calvin, 'Pouring a Healing Oil Over Troubled Waters.' *Australian Doctor*, 7 August, 1984. pp.14–15.

Olsol, A. & Farrar Jr., G.E., 'Cajeput Oil,' *Dispensatory of the United States*, 25th ed., 1955.

Pena, Eduardo F., 'Melaleuca Alternifolio Oil — Its Use for Trichomonal Vaginitis and Other Vaginal Infections.' *Obstetrics and Gynecology*, June 1962. pp.793–5.

Penfold, Arthur R. & Morrison F.R., 'Australian Tea Trees of Economic Value', *Technological Museum Bulletin*, No.14. 1929.

Penfold, Arthur R. & Morrison F.R., 'Some Notes of the Essential Oil of Melaleuca Alternifolia', *Australian Journal of Pharmacy*, 30 March, 1937, pp.274.

Penfold, A., '*Melaleuca alternifolia* (Cheel)', *Journal of the Royal Society of New South Wales*, 59:318, 1925.

Poucher, W.A., 'Tea Tree Oil', *Perfumes, Cosmetics and Soap*, 4th ed. 1:370, 1936.

Walker, Morton, 'Clinical Investigation of Australian *Melaleuca Alternifolia* for a Variety of Common Foot Problems.' *Current Podiatry*, April 1972.

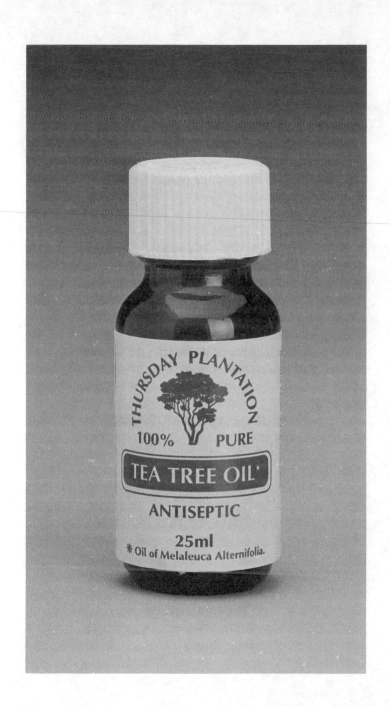

Where to obtain Tea Tree Oil

In the U.K.

Illingworth Health Foods,
York House,
York Street,
Bradford, BB8 0HR

Illingworth Health Foods distribute to well over a thousand health food shops, one of which may well be in your area.

In the U.S.A. and Canada

Thursday Plantation, Inc.,
South Coast Business Park,
6440-B Via Real,
Carpinteria,
California, CA 93013

Elsewhere

Thursday Plantation
Head Office,
Pacific Highway,
Ballina, N.S.W., 2378
Australia